Omega 3 Diet Guide for Beginners

The Importance of Omega 3 in Diet

By

Dougal Ewen

Copyright@2024

Table of Contents

CHAPTER 1

Introduction to Omega 3 Diet

1.1 What are Omega 3 Fatty Acids?

Omega-3 fatty acids are a family of essential polyunsaturated fats that play crucial roles in human health. They are called "essential" because the human body cannot synthesize them on its own, so they must be obtained through dietary sources. These fats are vital for various bodily functions, including but not limited to brain development, heart health, immune function, and inflammation regulation.

Chemically, omega-3 fatty acids are characterized by the presence of a double bond located three carbon atoms away from the methyl end of their carbon chain. This structural feature differentiates them from omega-6 fatty acids, another essential fatty acid group, which has a double bond six carbons away from the methyl end.

The primary types of omega-3 fatty acids include alpha-linolenic acid (ALA), eicosapentaenoic acid (EPA), and docosahexaenoic acid (DHA). ALA is predominantly found in plant-based sources such as flaxseeds, chia seeds, and walnuts. EPA and DHA, on the other hand, are mainly obtained from marine sources like fatty fish (salmon, mackerel, sardines), algae, and fish oil supplements.

Each type of omega-3 fatty acid serves distinct functions within the body. ALA, for instance, is converted to EPA and DHA in small amounts in the body, although this conversion process is not highly efficient. EPA and DHA, found predominantly in marine sources, are directly utilized by the body and are particularly important for maintaining cardiovascular health, supporting brain function, and promoting overall well-being.

Research indicates that omega-3 fatty acids offer a myriad of health benefits. They are known for their anti-inflammatory properties, which can help reduce the risk of chronic diseases such as heart disease, arthritis, and certain types of cancer. Additionally, omega-3s are crucial for cognitive function and may play a role in mood regulation, making them essential for mental health.

In recent years, the importance of omega-3 fatty acids in the diet has gained significant attention, leading to increased consumption through dietary modifications and supplementation. Health organizations and experts often recommend incorporating omega-3-rich foods into daily meals or considering supplementation, especially for individuals who may not consume adequate amounts through diet alone.

omega-3 fatty acids are essential nutrients with diverse physiological functions and numerous health benefits. Understanding their role in the body and incorporating them into a balanced diet can contribute to overall health and well-being.

1.2 Importance of Omega 3 in Diet

The importance of omega-3 fatty acids in the diet cannot be overstated due to their critical roles in maintaining optimal health and well-being. Here are several key reasons highlighting the significance of omega-3s:

1. **Brain Health and Development**: Omega-3 fatty acids, particularly EPA and DHA, are fundamental building blocks for brain tissue

and play a crucial role in brain development and function. They are highly concentrated in the brain and are essential for cognitive function, memory, and learning throughout all stages of life. Adequate intake of omega-3s, especially during pregnancy and early childhood, is associated with better neurodevelopment and cognitive outcomes.

2. **Heart Health**: Omega-3 fatty acids have been extensively studied for their cardiovascular benefits. They help maintain healthy cholesterol levels by reducing triglycerides and increasing high-density lipoprotein (HDL) cholesterol. Additionally, omega-3s have anti-inflammatory properties that can help reduce inflammation in blood vessels, lower blood pressure, and

decrease the risk of heart disease, heart attacks, and strokes.

3. **Inflammation Regulation**: Chronic inflammation is linked to the development of various diseases, including cardiovascular disease, arthritis, and metabolic syndrome. Omega-3 fatty acids, particularly EPA and DHA, have potent anti-inflammatory effects that can help modulate the body's inflammatory response. By reducing inflammation, omega-3s may help mitigate the risk and severity of inflammatory conditions.

4. **Eye Health**: DHA, one of the primary omega-3 fatty acids, is a major component of the retina in the eye. Adequate intake of DHA is crucial for maintaining optimal eye health, particularly for visual development in infants and the prevention of age-related macular

degeneration and other eye conditions in adults.

5. **Joint Health**: Omega-3 fatty acids have been shown to have beneficial effects on joint health, particularly in individuals with rheumatoid arthritis and osteoarthritis. They help reduce joint pain, stiffness, and inflammation, potentially improving overall joint function and mobility.

6. **Mood and Mental Health**: Omega-3 fatty acids play a role in regulating neurotransmitter function and may have antidepressant and mood-stabilizing effects. Research suggests that supplementation with omega-3s, especially EPA, may help alleviate symptoms of depression, anxiety, and other mood disorders.

7. **Skin Health**: Omega-3 fatty acids are essential for maintaining healthy skin cell membranes and promoting moisture retention. They also have anti-inflammatory properties that may help manage skin conditions such as eczema, psoriasis, and acne.

8. **Overall Well-being**: Incorporating omega-3-rich foods into the diet or supplementing with omega-3 fatty acids can contribute to overall health and well-being. From supporting cellular function to promoting immune health, omega-3s play diverse roles in maintaining optimal physiological function and enhancing quality of life.

Omega-3 fatty acids are indispensable nutrients that are vital for various aspects of health, including brain function, heart health, inflammation regulation, and overall well-being. Ensuring an adequate intake of omega-3s through diet or supplementation is essential for optimizing health outcomes and reducing the risk of chronic diseases.

CHAPTER 2

Types of Omega 3 Fatty Acids

2.1 Alpha-Linolenic Acid (ALA)

Alpha-linolenic acid (ALA) is a short-chain omega-3 fatty acid that is predominantly found in plant-based sources such as flaxseeds, chia seeds, hemp seeds, walnuts, and soybeans. It is considered an essential fatty acid because the human body cannot synthesize it and must obtain it through dietary sources. ALA serves as a precursor to the long-chain omega-3 fatty acids, eicosapentaenoic acid (EPA), and docosahexaenoic acid (DHA). While ALA provides some health benefits on its own, its primary importance lies in its conversion to EPA and DHA, albeit this conversion is limited in efficiency.

2.2 Eicosapentaenoic Acid (EPA)

Eicosapentaenoic acid (EPA) is a long-chain omega-3 fatty acid found primarily in marine sources such as fatty fish (e.g., salmon, mackerel, tuna, herring) and seafood. EPA is synthesized from alpha-linolenic acid (ALA) in the body, although this conversion process is not highly efficient. EPA plays crucial roles in cardiovascular health, inflammation regulation, and mood modulation. It is particularly known for its anti-inflammatory properties, which contribute to its cardiovascular benefits and its potential therapeutic effects on conditions such as rheumatoid arthritis and depression.

2.3 Docosahexaenoic Acid (DHA)

Docosahexaenoic acid (DHA) is another long-chain omega-3 fatty acid predominantly found in marine sources such as fatty fish, algae, and fish oil supplements. DHA is essential for brain health, particularly during fetal development and infancy, where it plays a critical role in neural and visual development. It is a major component of the brain and retina and is important for cognitive function, memory, and learning throughout life. DHA also supports cardiovascular health, eye health, and may have anti-inflammatory effects similar to EPA.

The three main types of omega-3 fatty acids—alpha-linolenic acid (ALA), eicosapentaenoic acid (EPA), and docosahexaenoic acid (DHA)—each have unique roles and sources in the diet. While ALA is primarily found in plant-based sources and serves as a precursor to EPA and DHA, EPA and DHA are predominantly obtained from marine sources and play essential roles in cardiovascular health, brain function, inflammation regulation, and overall well-being.

CHAPTER 3

Food Sources of Omega

3.1 Fatty Fish

Fatty fish are among the richest dietary sources of omega-3 fatty acids, particularly eicosapentaenoic acid (EPA) and docosahexaenoic acid (DHA). These fish accumulate omega-3s by consuming algae and other marine organisms that produce these essential fatty acids. Including fatty fish in your diet regularly can significantly boost your omega-3 intake. Some common examples of fatty fish include:

- Salmon: Salmon is one of the most popular and widely consumed fatty fish. It is rich in both EPA and DHA, making it an excellent choice for obtaining omega-3s. Wild-caught salmon generally contains higher levels of omega-3s compared to farm-raised salmon.

- Mackerel: Mackerel is another oily fish that is packed with omega-3 fatty acids. It is particularly high in both EPA and DHA, providing a substantial portion of your daily omega-3 requirements.

- Sardines: Sardines are small, oily fish that are often enjoyed canned. They are an affordable and convenient way to incorporate omega-3s into your diet. Sardines contain significant amounts of EPA and DHA, along with other essential nutrients like calcium and vitamin D.

- Trout: Trout is a freshwater fish that is also rich in omega-3 fatty acids. Rainbow trout, in particular, is known for its high omega-3 content, making it a nutritious choice for those seeking to increase their intake of these beneficial fats.

- Herring: Herring is another oily fish that is commonly consumed for its omega-3 content. It is often smoked, pickled, or canned and can be enjoyed in various dishes such as salads, sandwiches, or as a standalone protein source.

Incorporating fatty fish into your diet at least two to three times per week can help ensure an adequate intake of omega-3 fatty acids. However, it's essential to be mindful of the mercury content in certain types of fish, especially for pregnant women, nursing mothers, and young children. Opting for smaller fish varieties and choosing wild-caught options can help minimize exposure to environmental contaminants while still reaping the benefits of omega-3-rich seafood.

3.2 Plant-Based Sources

While fatty fish are the most well-known sources of omega-3 fatty acids, there are also several plant-based sources that provide alpha-linolenic acid (ALA), a precursor to EPA and DHA. Incorporating these plant-based foods into your diet can help boost your omega-3 intake, particularly for individuals following vegetarian or vegan diets. Some common plant-based sources of omega-3s include:

- Flaxseeds: Flaxseeds are one of the richest plant-based sources of ALA. They can be ground and added to smoothies, yogurt, oatmeal, or baked goods to increase your omega-3 intake. Flaxseed oil is another option, although it lacks the fiber content of whole flaxseeds.

- Chia Seeds: Chia seeds are tiny seeds that are packed with omega-

3 fatty acids, fiber, and various other nutrients. They can be soaked in liquid to form a gel-like consistency and used as a thickening agent in puddings, smoothies, or overnight oats.

- Hemp Seeds: Hemp seeds are a nutritious source of omega-3s, protein, and healthy fats. They can be sprinkled on salads, yogurt, or cereal, or incorporated into homemade energy bars or granola.

- Walnuts: Walnuts are one of the few tree nuts that contain significant amounts of ALA. They make for a convenient and portable snack and can also be added to salads, oatmeal, or baked goods for a nutritional boost.

- Soybeans and Soy Products: Soybeans and soy products like tofu, tempeh, and edamame are rich in ALA and can be incorporated into a variety of dishes as a plant-based protein source.

- Brussels Sprouts: Brussels sprouts are a cruciferous vegetable that contains ALA. They can be roasted, steamed, or sautéed and enjoyed as a side dish or added to salads and stir-fries.

By including a variety of these plant-based sources of omega-3s in your diet, you can help ensure that you're meeting your body's needs for these essential fatty acids, even if you don't consume fish.

3.3 Supplements

In addition to obtaining omega-3 fatty acids from food sources, some individuals may choose to take omega-3 supplements to ensure an adequate intake, particularly if they have specific dietary restrictions or preferences. Omega-3 supplements typically come in the form of fish oil, krill oil, or algae oil, which provide EPA and DHA directly.

- Fish Oil Supplements: Fish oil supplements are derived from the tissues of fatty fish and contain concentrated amounts of EPA and DHA. They come in liquid or capsule form and are widely available over-the-counter.

- Krill Oil Supplements: Krill oil is extracted from tiny shrimp-like crustaceans called krill. It is rich in EPA and DHA and is often marketed as having superior absorption compared to fish oil.

- Algae Oil Supplements: Algae oil supplements are a vegan-friendly alternative to fish oil, as they are derived from algae, which is the primary source of EPA and DHA in the marine food chain. These supplements provide a direct source of omega-3 fatty acids without the need for fish-derived ingredients.

Supplementation with omega-3 fatty acids may be beneficial for individuals who have difficulty obtaining sufficient amounts through diet alone, such as those who dislike or cannot consume fish, or those with certain medical conditions. However, it's essential to consult with a healthcare professional before starting any supplementation regimen to determine the appropriate dosage and ensure it is safe and suitable for your individual needs.

CHAPTER 4

Health Benefits of Omega-3 Diet

4.1 Heart Health

Omega-3 fatty acids, particularly eicosapentaenoic acid (EPA) and docosahexaenoic acid (DHA), have long been recognized for their profound benefits on heart health. Incorporating omega-3-rich foods into the diet or supplementing with omega-3 fatty acids has been associated with several cardioprotective effects, including:

- **Reduced Triglyceride Levels**: Omega-3s can lower triglyceride levels, a type of fat in the bloodstream that, when elevated, increases the risk of heart disease.

- **Improved Lipid Profile**: Omega-3s can increase levels of high-density lipoprotein (HDL) cholesterol, often referred to as "good" cholesterol, while decreasing levels of low-density lipoprotein (LDL) cholesterol, or "bad" cholesterol, thus promoting a healthier lipid profile.

- **Blood Pressure Regulation**: Omega-3s have mild blood pressure-lowering effects, which can help reduce the risk of hypertension and cardiovascular events like heart attacks and strokes.

- **Anti-inflammatory Properties**: Omega-3 fatty acids possess anti-inflammatory properties, which can help reduce inflammation in blood vessels and decrease the risk of atherosclerosis, a condition characterized by the buildup of plaque in the arteries.

- **Prevention of Arrhythmias**: Omega-3s may help prevent irregular heartbeats (arrhythmias) and reduce the risk of sudden cardiac death, particularly in individuals with a history of heart disease.

Diet rich in omega-3 fatty acids, along with other heart-healthy lifestyle practices such as regular physical activity and maintaining a healthy weight, can contribute to better cardiovascular health and a reduced risk of heart disease.

4.2 Brain Health

Omega-3 fatty acids are essential for optimal brain health and function throughout all stages of life. They play crucial roles in neurodevelopment during infancy and childhood, and they continue to support cognitive function and mental well-being in adulthood and old age.

Some key benefits of omega-3s for brain health include:

- **Brain Development**: DHA, in particular, is a major structural component of the brain and is essential for proper brain development during fetal development and infancy. Adequate intake of omega-3s during pregnancy and breastfeeding is associated with better cognitive outcomes in children.

- **Cognitive Function**: Omega-3 fatty acids are important for maintaining cognitive function, memory, and attention as we age. They may help protect against age-related cognitive decline and reduce the risk of neurodegenerative diseases such as Alzheimer's disease and dementia.

- **Mood Regulation**: EPA, in particular, has been shown to have mood-stabilizing and antidepressant effects. Omega-3 supplementation may help alleviate symptoms of depression, anxiety, and other mood disorders.

- **Neuroprotection**: Omega-3s have antioxidant and anti-inflammatory properties that can help protect brain cells from damage and promote neuroplasticity, the brain's ability to adapt and form new connections.

Incorporating omega-3-rich foods into the diet or taking omega-3 supplements may help support overall brain health and cognitive function, leading to improved mental well-being and quality of life.

4.3 Eye Health

Omega-3 fatty acids, particularly DHA, are essential for maintaining optimal eye health, particularly the health of the retina, which is the light-sensitive tissue lining the back of the eye. Some key benefits of omega-3s for eye health include:

- **Visual Development**: DHA is a major structural component of the retina, especially during fetal development and infancy. Adequate intake of omega-3s during pregnancy and breastfeeding is crucial for normal visual development in infants.

- **Prevention of Age-Related Macular Degeneration (AMD)**: AMD is a leading cause of vision loss in older adults. Omega-3 fatty acids have been shown to reduce the risk of AMD and slow its progression by protecting retinal cells from oxidative damage and inflammation.

- **Dry Eye Syndrome**: Omega-3 supplementation may help alleviate symptoms of dry eye syndrome, a common condition characterized by dryness, irritation, and discomfort in the eyes. Omega-3s help maintain tear film integrity and reduce inflammation on the ocular surface.

Incorporating omega-3-rich foods into the diet, such as fatty fish, flaxseeds, and walnuts, can support overall eye health and may help reduce the risk of age-related eye diseases.

4.4 Inflammation Reduction

Chronic inflammation is a common underlying factor in many chronic diseases, including cardiovascular disease, diabetes, arthritis, and certain types of cancer. Omega-3 fatty acids, particularly EPA and DHA, possess potent anti-inflammatory properties that can help modulate the body's inflammatory response and reduce the risk of inflammation-related diseases. Some key ways in which omega-3s can help reduce inflammation include:

- **Inhibition of Pro-inflammatory Pathways**: Omega-3 fatty acids compete with omega-6 fatty acids, which are pro-inflammatory, for incorporation into cell membranes. By increasing the ratio of omega-3s to omega-6s, omega-3s help dampen inflammatory responses in the body.

- **Decreased Production of Inflammatory Mediators**: EPA and DHA can inhibit the production of pro-inflammatory cytokines, chemokines, and other inflammatory mediators, thereby reducing systemic inflammation and its detrimental effects on tissues and organs.

- **Resolution of Inflammation**: Omega-3 fatty acids promote the resolution of inflammation by stimulating the production of specialized pro-resolving mediators (SPMs) that help resolve inflammatory responses and restore tissue homeostasis.

Incorporating omega-3-rich foods into the diet or taking omega-3 supplements can help mitigate chronic inflammation and reduce the risk of inflammation-related diseases. However, it's essential to maintain a balanced ratio of omega-3 to omega-6 fatty acids and adopt other anti-inflammatory lifestyle practices, such as regular exercise, stress management, and a healthy diet rich in fruits, vegetables, and whole grains, for optimal inflammatory control and overall health.

4.5 Other Potential Benefits

While the health benefits of omega-3 fatty acids are well-established for heart health, brain health, eye health, and inflammation reduction, ongoing research suggests that omega-3s may offer additional advantages for overall well-being and disease prevention. Some other potential benefits of including omega-3-rich foods in the diet or supplementing with omega-3 fatty acids include:

1. **Bone Health**: Emerging evidence suggests that omega-3 fatty acids may play a role in promoting bone health and reducing the risk of osteoporosis. Omega-3s may help enhance bone mineral density and reduce bone loss by modulating inflammatory pathways and

promoting optimal calcium absorption and utilization.

2. **Muscle Recovery and Performance**: Omega-3 fatty acids may have benefits for athletes and individuals engaged in physical activity. Studies suggest that omega-3 supplementation may help reduce exercise-induced muscle soreness and inflammation, enhance muscle recovery, and improve overall exercise performance and endurance.

3. **Skin Health**: Omega-3 fatty acids are important for maintaining healthy skin cell membranes and promoting skin hydration and elasticity. Omega-3s may help improve various skin conditions, including eczema, psoriasis, acne, and premature aging, by reducing inflammation, supporting skin

barrier function, and promoting
wound healing.

4. **Metabolic Health**: Omega-3 fatty
   acids may have beneficial effects
   on metabolic health and insulin
   sensitivity, which are important
   for preventing and managing type
   2 diabetes and metabolic
   syndrome. Omega-3s may help
   regulate glucose metabolism,
   reduce insulin resistance, and
   improve lipid profile, contributing
   to better glycemic control and
   reduced risk of diabetes-related
   complications.

5. **Immune Function**: Omega-3
   fatty acids play a role in
   modulating immune function and
   promoting immune system
   balance. EPA and DHA have anti-
   inflammatory and
   immunomodulatory effects that
   may help regulate immune
   responses, reduce excessive

inflammation, and enhance immune cell function, thereby supporting overall immune health and resilience to infections.

Further research is needed to fully elucidate the extent of these potential benefits and their mechanisms of action, incorporating omega-3-rich foods into the diet or supplementing with omega-3 fatty acids may offer a multifaceted approach to promoting overall health and reducing the risk of various chronic diseases. However, it's important to consult with a healthcare professional before starting any new supplementation regimen, especially for individuals with pre-existing medical conditions or those taking medications, to ensure safety and efficacy.

CHAPTER 5

Omega 3 Diet and Chronic Diseases

5.1 Cardiovascular Disease

Cardiovascular disease (CVD) is a leading cause of morbidity and mortality worldwide, encompassing conditions such as coronary artery disease, heart failure, stroke, and peripheral artery disease. Omega-3 fatty acids, particularly eicosapentaenoic acid (EPA) and docosahexaenoic acid (DHA), have been extensively studied for their potential protective effects against cardiovascular disease. Here's how omega-3s may impact various aspects of cardiovascular health:

- **Reduced Risk of Coronary Heart Disease (CHD)**: Numerous observational studies and clinical trials have suggested that regular consumption of omega-3-rich foods or supplementation with omega-3 fatty acids is associated with a lower risk of coronary heart disease. Omega-3s can help reduce triglyceride levels, improve lipid profiles by increasing high-density lipoprotein (HDL) cholesterol and reducing low-density lipoprotein (LDL) cholesterol, and decrease the risk of plaque buildup in the arteries (atherosclerosis), thus lowering the risk of heart attacks and other cardiovascular events.

- **Antiarrhythmic Effects**: Omega-3 fatty acids have antiarrhythmic properties, meaning they can help stabilize heart rhythm and reduce the risk of potentially life-threatening arrhythmias, such as ventricular fibrillation and sudden cardiac death. EPA and DHA can modulate ion channel function, reduce myocardial excitability, and improve electrical stability in the heart, thereby lowering the incidence of arrhythmias.

- **Blood Pressure Regulation**: Omega-3 fatty acids have mild blood pressure-lowering effects, which can help reduce hypertension and lower the risk of cardiovascular complications such as stroke and heart failure. EPA and DHA can dilate blood vessels, improve endothelial function, and inhibit the production of vasoconstrictive substances, contributing to better blood pressure control.

- **Anti-inflammatory Effects**: Chronic inflammation plays a key role in the development and progression of cardiovascular disease. Omega-3 fatty acids possess potent anti-inflammatory properties that can help modulate inflammatory pathways, reduce vascular inflammation, and mitigate the inflammatory processes underlying atherosclerosis and other cardiovascular conditions.

- **Endothelial Function Improvement**: Omega-3 fatty acids can improve endothelial function, which refers to the ability of blood vessels to dilate and constrict in response to various stimuli. EPA and DHA promote the production of nitric oxide, a vasodilator that helps regulate blood flow and vascular tone, thereby enhancing endothelial-dependent vasodilation and vascular health.

Overall, incorporating omega-3-rich foods into the diet or supplementing with omega-3 fatty acids may help reduce the risk of cardiovascular disease, improve lipid profiles, stabilize heart rhythm, lower blood pressure, and mitigate inflammation, thus promoting better cardiovascular health and reducing the burden of cardiovascular morbidity and mortality. However, it's important to maintain a balanced diet, engage in regular physical activity, and adopt other heart-healthy lifestyle practices for optimal cardiovascular risk reduction. Individuals with pre-existing cardiovascular conditions or those at high risk for CVD should consult with a healthcare professional for personalized recommendations regarding omega-3 supplementation and cardiovascular disease prevention strategies.

5.2 Cognitive Decline and Neurological Disorders

Cognitive decline and neurological disorders, including Alzheimer's disease, dementia, Parkinson's disease, and multiple sclerosis, present significant challenges to individuals and their families, as well as to healthcare systems globally. Research suggests that omega-3 fatty acids may play a beneficial role in maintaining brain health and reducing the risk of cognitive decline and certain neurological disorders. Here's how omega-3s may impact cognitive function and neurological health:

- **Neurodevelopment**: Omega-3 fatty acids, particularly docosahexaenoic acid (DHA), are critical for brain development during fetal development and infancy. Adequate intake of omega-3s during pregnancy and breastfeeding is associated with better cognitive outcomes in children, including improved attention, memory, and language development.

- **Cognitive Function**: Omega-3 fatty acids are important for

maintaining cognitive function
and mental acuity throughout life.
Epidemiological studies have
suggested that higher intake of
omega-3-rich foods or
supplementation with omega-3
fatty acids is associated with
better cognitive performance,
reduced risk of cognitive decline,
and lower incidence of age-related
cognitive impairment.

- **Neuroprotection**: Omega-3 fatty
acids possess neuroprotective
properties that can help protect
against neuronal damage and
promote neuronal survival. EPA
and DHA can modulate
inflammatory pathways, reduce
oxidative stress, and enhance
synaptic plasticity, thereby
mitigating neuronal dysfunction
and degeneration associated with
neurodegenerative diseases.

- **Alzheimer's Disease and Dementia**: Several studies have suggested that omega-3 fatty acids may help reduce the risk of Alzheimer's disease and dementia and slow the progression of cognitive decline in individuals with mild cognitive impairment. EPA and DHA can help reduce the formation of beta-amyloid plaques and tau protein tangles, which are hallmark pathological features of Alzheimer's disease.

- **Parkinson's Disease**: Preliminary research indicates that omega-3 fatty acids may have neuroprotective effects against Parkinson's disease, a progressive neurodegenerative disorder characterized by the loss of dopamine-producing neurons in the brain. Omega-3s may help enhance dopamine transmission, reduce neuroinflammation, and promote neuronal survival in Parkinson's disease models.

- **Multiple Sclerosis (MS)**: Omega-3 fatty acids may have potential benefits for individuals with multiple sclerosis, an autoimmune disorder that affects the central nervous system. EPA and DHA can help modulate immune responses, reduce neuroinflammation, and promote remyelination, which may help alleviate symptoms and slow disease progression in MS patients.

While further research is needed to elucidate the precise mechanisms underlying the effects of omega-3 fatty acids on cognitive function and neurological health, current evidence suggests that incorporating omega-3-rich foods into the diet or supplementing with omega-3 fatty acids may offer potential benefits for maintaining brain health, reducing the risk of cognitive decline, and mitigating the progression of certain neurological disorders. However, it's important to consult with a healthcare professional before starting any new supplementation regimen, especially for individuals with pre-existing neurological conditions or those taking medications, to ensure safety and efficacy.

5.3 Arthritis and Joint Health

Arthritis, a condition characterized by inflammation and stiffness of the joints, affects millions of people worldwide and can significantly impact quality of life. Omega-3 fatty acids have been studied for their potential anti-inflammatory effects and their role in managing symptoms associated with various forms of arthritis, including rheumatoid arthritis (RA), osteoarthritis (OA), and other inflammatory joint conditions. Here's how omega-3s may impact arthritis and joint health:

- **Anti-inflammatory Properties**: Omega-3 fatty acids, particularly eicosapentaenoic acid (EPA) and docosahexaenoic acid (DHA), possess potent anti-inflammatory properties that can help mitigate inflammation in the joints and reduce pain, stiffness, and swelling associated with arthritis. EPA and DHA compete with arachidonic acid, an omega-6 fatty acid precursor of pro-inflammatory mediators, for incorporation into cell membranes, thereby reducing the production of inflammatory cytokines and eicosanoids.

- **Rheumatoid Arthritis (RA)**: Rheumatoid arthritis is an autoimmune disorder characterized by chronic

inflammation of the synovial
lining of the joints, leading to
joint damage and deformity.
Omega-3 fatty acids have been
shown to help alleviate symptoms
of RA, including joint pain,
morning stiffness, and
tender/swollen joints. EPA and
DHA can modulate immune
responses, reduce pro-
inflammatory cytokines, and
inhibit the activity of enzymes
involved in cartilage degradation
and bone resorption, thus slowing
disease progression and
preserving joint function.

- **Osteoarthritis (OA):**
  Osteoarthritis is a degenerative
  joint disease characterized by the
  breakdown of cartilage and the
  formation of bone spurs in the
  joints. While OA is primarily a
  mechanical and age-related
  condition, inflammation also

plays a role in its pathogenesis. Omega-3 fatty acids may help reduce inflammation and slow the progression of OA by inhibiting cartilage degradation, promoting cartilage repair, and reducing pain and disability associated with the disease.

- **Other Inflammatory Joint Conditions**: Omega-3 fatty acids may also benefit individuals with other inflammatory joint conditions, such as psoriatic arthritis, ankylosing spondylitis, and juvenile idiopathic arthritis. EPA and DHA can help modulate immune responses, decrease inflammatory markers, and improve overall joint health and function in these conditions.

- **Pain Relief**: Omega-3 fatty acids may help alleviate joint pain and improve mobility in individuals with arthritis. EPA and DHA have been shown to have analgesic effects, reducing the need for nonsteroidal anti-inflammatory drugs (NSAIDs) and other pain medications in some cases.

Incorporating omega-3-rich foods into the diet or supplementing with omega-3 fatty acids may help reduce inflammation, alleviate symptoms, and improve joint health and function in individuals with arthritis and other inflammatory joint conditions. However, it's important to consult with a healthcare professional before starting any new supplementation regimen, especially for individuals with pre-existing joint conditions or those taking medications, to ensure safety and efficacy. Additionally, omega-3 supplementation should be combined with other arthritis management strategies, such as exercise, weight management, and joint protection techniques, for optimal symptom relief and disease management.

CHAPTER 6

Implementing an Omega 3 Diet

6.1 Cooking and Preparation Tips

Incorporating omega-3-rich foods into your diet can be delicious and easy with the right cooking and preparation techniques. Here are some tips to help you maximize the omega-3 content of your meals:

- **Choose Fatty Fish**: Opt for fatty fish such as salmon, mackerel, sardines, trout, and herring, which are among the richest sources of omega-3 fatty acids. When selecting fish, aim for wild-caught varieties whenever possible, as they tend to have higher omega-3 content than farm-raised fish.

- **Grill or Bake**: Grill, bake, or broil fish instead of frying to retain the omega-3 fatty acids and minimize added fats. Season fish with herbs, spices, and citrus for added flavor without extra calories.

- **Include Plant-Based Sources**: Incorporate plant-based sources of omega-3s such as flaxseeds, chia seeds, hemp seeds, walnuts, and soybeans into your meals. Add ground flaxseeds or chia seeds to smoothies, yogurt, oatmeal, or baked goods. Sprinkle hemp seeds or chopped walnuts on salads, soups, or stir-fries. Use tofu or tempeh in stir-fries, curries, or salads for a plant-based protein option.

- **Use Healthy Oils**: Cook with oils rich in alpha-linolenic acid (ALA), such as flaxseed oil, hempseed oil, or canola oil, to boost your omega-3 intake. Use these oils in salad dressings, dips, marinades, or as a finishing oil for cooked dishes.

- **Limit Processing**: Minimize processing and cooking times to preserve the omega-3 content of foods. Overcooking or prolonged heating can degrade omega-3 fatty acids, so aim for shorter cooking times and gentler cooking methods whenever possible.

- **Supplement Wisely**: If you have difficulty meeting your omega-3 needs through diet alone, consider taking omega-3 supplements under the guidance of a healthcare professional. Choose high-quality supplements that contain EPA and DHA in bioavailable forms and follow the recommended dosage instructions.

Variety of omega-3-rich foods into your diet and using healthy cooking and preparation methods, you can enjoy the nutritional benefits of omega 3 fatty acids while savoring delicious and nourishing meals. Remember to prioritize whole, minimally processed foods and consult with a registered dietitian or healthcare provider for personalized dietary recommendations based on your individual needs and preferences.

6.2 Balancing Omega 3 with Omega 6

Achieving a healthy balance between omega-3 and omega-6 fatty acids is essential for optimal health, as both types of fatty acids play important roles in the body. However, modern Western diets often contain an imbalance, with an overabundance of omega-6 fatty acids relative to omega-3s. This imbalance has been associated with increased inflammation and the development of chronic diseases. Here are some tips for balancing omega-3 and omega-6 fatty acids in your diet:

1. **Increase Omega-3 Intake**: Focus on increasing your intake of omega-3-rich foods, such as fatty fish (salmon, mackerel, sardines), flaxseeds, chia seeds, walnuts, and hemp seeds. Aim to include these foods in your diet regularly to boost your omega-3 levels.

2. **Limit Omega-6-Rich Foods**: Be mindful of sources of omega-6 fatty acids in your diet, such as processed vegetable oils (soybean oil, corn oil, sunflower oil, safflower oil), fried foods, and processed snacks and baked goods. These foods are commonly

found in fast food, packaged snacks, and convenience foods. Limiting your intake of these foods can help reduce your overall omega-6 consumption.

3. **Choose Healthy Cooking Oils**: Opt for cooking oils that are lower in omega-6 fatty acids and higher in monounsaturated fats or omega-3 fatty acids, such as olive oil, avocado oil, or canola oil. These oils are more stable at high temperatures and can help balance your omega-6 intake.

4. **Read Food Labels**: Pay attention to food labels when purchasing packaged and processed foods. Check the ingredient list for sources of omega-6 fatty acids, such as soybean oil or corn oil, and choose products with healthier fat sources whenever possible.

5. **Eat Whole Foods**: Focus on consuming whole, minimally processed foods that naturally contain a balanced ratio of omega-3 to omega-6 fatty acids. Whole grains, legumes, fruits, and vegetables are excellent sources of nutrients and provide a healthier balance of fats compared to processed foods.

6. **Consider Omega-3 Supplements**: If you struggle to obtain sufficient omega-3 fatty acids from dietary sources alone, consider taking omega-3 supplements to help rebalance your omega-3 to omega-6 ratio. Look for supplements that contain both EPA and DHA in bioavailable forms, and consult with a healthcare professional for personalized recommendations.

7. **Track Your Intake**: Keep track of your omega-3 and omega-6

intake using a food diary or nutrition tracking app. This can help you become more aware of your dietary patterns and make adjustments to achieve a healthier balance of fats.

Focusing on increasing omega-3 intake, limiting omega-6-rich foods, choosing healthier cooking oils, eating whole foods, and considering supplementation, if necessary, you can achieve a better balance of omega-3 and omega-6 fatty acids in your diet. This balanced approach can help support overall health and reduce the risk of inflammation-related chronic diseases.

CHAPTER 7

Risks and Considerations

7.1 Mercury Contamination in Fish

While fatty fish are excellent sources of omega-3 fatty acids, they may also contain varying levels of mercury, a toxic heavy metal that can have harmful effects on human health, particularly in high doses. Mercury accumulates in the tissues of fish over time, primarily through the food chain, and larger predatory fish tend to have higher levels of mercury due to biomagnification. Here are some considerations regarding mercury contamination in fish:

- **Health Risks**: Mercury exposure, especially methylmercury found in fish, can have adverse effects on the nervous system, cardiovascular system, kidneys, and reproductive system. In particular, mercury exposure during pregnancy can harm fetal development and lead to neurological deficits, cognitive impairments, and developmental delays in children.

- **High-Mercury Fish**: Certain species of fish are known to have higher levels of mercury and are recommended to be consumed in moderation, especially for vulnerable populations such as pregnant women, nursing mothers, young children, and individuals with compromised kidney function. Examples of high-mercury fish include shark, swordfish, king mackerel, and tilefish.

- **Low-Mercury Alternatives**: To minimize mercury exposure while still obtaining the health benefits of omega-3 fatty acids, consider choosing fish with lower mercury levels. Examples of low-mercury fish include salmon, trout, sardines, anchovies, and herring. These options are generally safer for regular consumption and provide ample omega-3s without significant mercury exposure.

- **Variety and Moderation**: Instead of relying on a single type of fish for omega-3s, aim to include a variety of seafood in your diet to reduce the risk of excessive mercury exposure. By rotating between different types of fish, you can enjoy the nutritional benefits of seafood while mitigating potential health risks associated with mercury contamination. Additionally, practice moderation in fish consumption and follow dietary guidelines regarding recommended servings per week to minimize mercury intake.

- **Safe Cooking Practices**: Proper cooking methods can help reduce mercury exposure in fish. Remove the skin and trim visible fat before cooking, as mercury tends to accumulate in these tissues. Additionally, choose cooking methods that allow excess fat to drip away, such as grilling, baking, or broiling, rather than frying, which can retain more contaminants.

- **Consultation with Healthcare Providers**: Pregnant women, nursing mothers, and individuals with specific health concerns should consult with their healthcare providers for personalized recommendations regarding fish consumption and omega-3 supplementation. Healthcare professionals can provide guidance on safe fish choices, portion sizes, and supplementation to ensure optimal nutrition while minimizing mercury exposure.

while mercury contamination in fish is a valid concern, the health benefits of consuming omega-3-rich fish can outweigh the risks for most individuals when consumed in moderation and as part of a balanced diet. By making informed choices, practicing moderation, and seeking guidance from healthcare professionals, you can enjoy the nutritional benefits of fish while minimizing potential health risks associated with mercury contamination.

7.2 Potential Interactions with Medications

When incorporating omega-3 fatty acids into your diet or taking omega-3 supplements, it's essential to be aware of potential interactions with medications. Omega-3 fatty acids can affect the metabolism and efficacy of certain medications, leading to potential adverse effects or reduced therapeutic outcomes. Here are some considerations regarding potential interactions with medications:

- **Blood Thinners (Anticoagulants/Antiplatelet Drugs)**: Omega-3 fatty acids have blood-thinning properties and may enhance the effects of blood-thinning medications such as warfarin (Coumadin), clopidogrel (Plavix), aspirin, and other antiplatelet drugs. Concurrent use of omega-3 supplements with these medications may increase the risk of bleeding or bruising. It's important to consult with a healthcare professional before combining omega-3 supplements with blood thinners, as dosage adjustments may be necessary to prevent excessive bleeding.

- **Blood Pressure Medications**: Omega-3 fatty acids can modestly lower blood pressure, so caution should be exercised when combining omega-3 supplements with antihypertensive medications such as ACE inhibitors, beta-blockers, calcium channel blockers, or diuretics. Close monitoring of blood pressure is recommended, and dosage adjustments may be needed under the guidance of a healthcare provider.

- **Cholesterol-Lowering Drugs (Statins)**: Omega-3 fatty acids may have synergistic effects with statin medications commonly used to lower cholesterol levels. However, combining omega-3 supplements with statins may increase the risk of muscle-related side effects, such as myalgia (muscle pain) or rhabdomyolysis (muscle breakdown). Healthcare professionals should monitor patients closely for potential adverse effects when combining omega-3 supplements with statin therapy.

- **Immunosuppressants**: Omega-3 fatty acids have anti-inflammatory properties and may interact with immunosuppressive medications used to treat autoimmune disorders or organ transplantation. Concurrent use of omega-3 supplements with immunosuppressants may enhance immunosuppression and increase the risk of infections or other complications. Healthcare providers should monitor patients closely and adjust medication doses as needed.

- **Other Medications**: Omega-3 fatty acids may interact with other medications or supplements, including nonsteroidal anti-inflammatory drugs (NSAIDs), corticosteroids, hormonal therapies, and herbal supplements. It's important to consult with a healthcare professional before combining omega-3 supplements with any medications or supplements to avoid potential interactions and ensure safety and efficacy.

Before starting any new supplementation regimen, especially if you are currently taking medications, it's crucial to discuss potential interactions with your healthcare provider. Healthcare professionals can provide personalized recommendations based on your medical history, current medications, and individual health needs to ensure safe and effective supplementation with omega-3 fatty acids.

7.3 Allergies and Sensitivities

Individuals with allergies or sensitivities to seafood, fish, or other sources of omega-3 fatty acids should exercise caution when incorporating omega-3-rich foods into their diet or taking omega-3 supplements. Here are some considerations regarding allergies and sensitivities:

- **Fish Allergies**: Fish allergies are relatively common and can range from mild to severe. Individuals with fish allergies should avoid consuming fish and fish-derived products, including fish oil supplements, to prevent allergic reactions. Instead, they can consider alternative sources of omega-3 fatty acids such as plant-based sources (flaxseeds, chia seeds, walnuts) or algae-based supplements, which are free from fish allergens.

- **Shellfish Allergies**: Some individuals may have allergies to shellfish, such as shrimp, crab, lobster, or mollusks. While fish oil supplements are generally free from shellfish allergens, it's essential to read product labels carefully and choose supplements from reputable manufacturers to minimize the risk of cross-contamination. Individuals with shellfish allergies should consult with their healthcare provider before starting any new supplements.

- **Cross-Reactivity**: Cross-reactivity between fish and other seafood allergens is possible, so individuals with fish allergies may also be at risk of allergic reactions to other types of seafood. It's important to be cautious when consuming seafood and to seek guidance from healthcare professionals if uncertain about potential allergens.

- **Plant-Based Alternatives**: For individuals with allergies or sensitivities to seafood, plant-based sources of omega-3 fatty acids can provide a safe alternative. Incorporating foods such as flaxseeds, chia seeds, hemp seeds, walnuts, and algae-based supplements into the diet can help meet omega-3 requirements without the risk of seafood allergies.

- **Consultation with Healthcare Providers**: Individuals with known allergies or sensitivities should consult with their healthcare providers or allergists for personalized recommendations regarding omega-3 supplementation and dietary choices. Healthcare professionals can help assess individual risk factors, provide guidance on allergen avoidance strategies, and recommend suitable alternatives to meet nutritional needs.

By being mindful of potential interactions with medications and allergies or sensitivities to seafood, individuals can safely incorporate omega-3 fatty acids into their diet or supplementation regimen while minimizing potential risks. It's important to seek guidance from healthcare professionals for personalized recommendations based on individual health status, medical history, and dietary preferences.

CHAPTER 8

Embracing an Omega-3 Diet

Incorporating omega-3 fatty acids into your diet can offer a wide range of health benefits, from supporting heart health and brain function to reducing inflammation and promoting overall well-being. Here are some tips for embracing an omega-3 diet and maximizing the nutritional benefits of these essential fatty acids:

1. **Eat Fatty Fish Regularly**: Make it a habit to include fatty fish such as salmon, mackerel, sardines, trout, and herring in your meals at least twice a week. These fish are rich sources of EPA and DHA, the two most beneficial forms of omega-3 fatty acids.

2. **Diversify Your Omega-3 Sources**: Don't limit yourself to just fish for omega-3s. Incorporate a variety of omega-3-rich foods into your diet, including plant-based sources such as flaxseeds, chia seeds, hemp seeds, walnuts, and algae-based supplements.

3. **Choose Whole Foods**: Focus on whole, minimally processed foods that naturally contain omega-3 fatty acids, rather than relying on supplements or fortified products. Whole foods provide a balanced array of nutrients and offer additional health benefits beyond just omega-3s.

4. **Opt for Healthy Cooking Methods**: When preparing omega-3-rich foods, choose healthy cooking methods such as grilling, baking, broiling, or steaming to preserve the

nutritional integrity of the ingredients. Avoid frying or deep-frying, as this can add unnecessary calories and unhealthy fats.

5. **Pair Omega-3s with Antioxidants**: Combine omega-3-rich foods with antioxidant-rich fruits, vegetables, herbs, and spices to enhance their health benefits. Antioxidants can help protect omega-3 fatty acids from oxidation and support overall cellular health.

6. **Be Mindful of Mercury**: While fish is an excellent source of omega-3s, be mindful of mercury contamination, especially in larger predatory fish. Choose fish lower in mercury and consider rotating between different types of seafood to minimize exposure.

7. **Read Labels**: When purchasing packaged or processed foods, read the ingredient labels carefully to identify sources of omega-3 fatty acids and ensure they are from reputable sources. Look for products made with natural, whole food ingredients whenever possible.

8. **Supplement Wisely**: If you're unable to meet your omega-3 needs through diet alone, consider supplementing with high-quality fish oil or algae-based omega-3 supplements. Choose supplements that provide a balanced ratio of EPA and DHA and are free from contaminants.

9. **Consult with a Healthcare Professional**: Before making any significant changes to your diet or starting a new supplementation regimen, consult with a healthcare professional or registered

dietitian. They can provide personalized recommendations based on your individual health status, dietary preferences, and nutritional needs.

10. **Make It Enjoyable**: Embracing an omega-3 diet doesn't have to be boring or restrictive. Get creative in the kitchen, experiment with new recipes, and find delicious ways to incorporate omega-3-rich foods into your meals. Enjoy the journey to better health and savor the nourishing benefits of omega-3 fatty acids in every bite.

11. **Share the Benefits**: Spread the word about the benefits of omega-3 fatty acids with friends, family, and loved ones. Encourage them to join you on your journey to better health by incorporating omega-3-rich foods into their diets or considering supplementation if needed.

Sharing knowledge and experiences can inspire others to make positive changes for their health as well.

12. **Stay Informed**: Stay up-to-date with the latest research and recommendations regarding omega-3 fatty acids and their impact on health. Science is constantly evolving, and new findings may emerge that further underscore the importance of omega-3s or provide insights into optimal dietary strategies. Keep an open mind and continue learning about how omega-3s can benefit your overall well-being.

13. **Monitor Your Progress**: Pay attention to how your body responds to your omega-3 diet. Keep track of any changes in your energy levels, mood, cognitive function, joint health, or other aspects of well-being. By

monitoring your progress, you can
adjust your dietary habits as
needed to optimize your health
and achieve your wellness goals.

14. **Seek Balance**: While omega-3
    fatty acids are important for
    health, they are just one
    component of a balanced diet and
    lifestyle. Aim for overall dietary
    balance by incorporating a variety
    of nutrient-rich foods, including
    fruits, vegetables, whole grains,
    lean proteins, and healthy fats.
    Balance your omega-3 intake with
    omega-6 and omega-9 fatty acids
    to maintain optimal health and
    support various bodily functions.

15. **Listen to Your Body**: Everyone's
    nutritional needs and preferences
    are unique. Pay attention to how
    different foods make you feel and
    adjust your dietary choices
    accordingly. If certain omega-3-
    rich foods don't agree with you or

you have specific dietary restrictions, explore alternative options that still provide essential nutrients and support your health goals.

16. **Stay Consistent**: Consistency is key when it comes to reaping the benefits of an omega-3 diet. Make omega-3-rich foods a regular part of your meals and aim for consistency in your dietary habits over time. Small, sustainable changes can lead to significant improvements in your health and well-being over the long term.

17. **Celebrate Successes**: Celebrate your successes along the way, no matter how small they may seem. Whether it's incorporating more omega-3-rich foods into your diet, achieving a health milestone, or simply feeling more energized and vibrant, take time to acknowledge and celebrate your

progress. Positive reinforcement can help keep you motivated and committed to your omega-3 journey.

18. **Stay Positive**: Embrace a positive mindset and focus on the benefits of nourishing your body with omega-3 fatty acids. Visualize yourself enjoying vibrant health, vitality, and well-being as you continue to prioritize your nutritional needs. A positive attitude can empower you to overcome challenges and stay on track toward achieving your health goals.

Incorporating these additional tips into your omega-3 journey, you can enhance the overall impact of your dietary choices and cultivate a healthier, more vibrant lifestyle.

9 798883 206626

COGNITIVE BEHAVIORAL THERAPY:

A Guide to Positive Psychology with Strategies & Techniques to Regain Happiness by Overcoming Anxiety, Depression, Negative Thought Patterns & Phobias

Larry Parsons

Table of Contents